Fabriane Sousa Araújo Lima
Antonio da Costa Cardoso Neto
Márcia Silva de Oliveira

NURSING ACTIONS

Fabriane Sousa Araújo Lima
Antonio da Costa Cardoso Neto
Márcia Silva de Oliveira

NURSING ACTIONS

IN BREAST CANCER PATIENTS

ScienciaScripts

This book is a translation from the original published under ISBN 978-620-6-76201-0.

Publisher:
Sciencia Scripts
is a trademark of
Dodo Books Indian Ocean Ltd. and OmniScriptum S.R.L publishing group

120 High Road, East Finchley, London, N2 9ED, United Kingdom
Str. Armeneasca 28/1, office 1, Chisinau MD-2012, Republic of Moldova, Europe
Printed at: see last page
ISBN: 978-620-8-13996-4

NURSING ACTIONS FOR BREAST CANCER PATIENTS

FABRIANE SOUSA ARAÚJO LIMA ANTONIO DA COSTA CARDOSO NETO MÁRCIA SILVA DE OLIVEIRA

NURSING CARE IS THE SCIENCE AND ART OF HUMAN CARE, ESSENTIAL FOR EVERYONE'S HEALTH AND WELL-BEING.

FLORENCE NIGHTINGALE

SUMMARY

1 INTRODUCTION

Breast carcinoma is the most prevalent neoplasm among women. According to global data from 2018, there were an estimated 2.1 million initial diagnoses of this pathology and 627,000 related deaths. In Brazil, 59,700 new diagnoses were expected in 2019, representing 29.5 per cent of all female malignant neoplasms, with a frequency of 56 cases per 100,000 inhabitants. In 2016, 16,069 women died from this type of cancer, making it the leading cause of death from neoplasms among women in Brazil (Silva et al., 2021).

Nursing intervention is essential at all stages faced by breast cancer (BC) patients, from prevention to treatment and subsequent recovery. Thus: "the nurse's role in the early detection of breast cancer is fundamental to stimulating women's adherence, including health promotion actions and even treatment and rehabilitation" (Teixeira et. al., 2017, p. 2). When it comes to diagnosing breast cancer, nurses are responsible for carrying out clinical examinations and observing premonitory symptoms. Their competence in detecting suspicious changes in the breasts is fundamental for referring patients for additional diagnostic procedures, such as mammography, ensuring early detection and effective treatment. During therapy for this disease, these professionals play a crucial role in the application of therapies and the control of adverse effects. In addition, nurses "work in the preoperative period for patients undergoing mastectomy, whether conservative or not. And [...] the needs of patients undergoing complementary treatment such as chemoprevention, radiotherapy and hormone therapy." (Mineo et. al., 2015, p. 2248) Nurses play a key role in encouraging adherence to treatment and providing emotional support for patients. Thanks to their close relationship with patients, they have the ability to assess the impact on the patient's health, taking into account not only physiological and clinical requirements, but also psychological and social demands.

The nursing team's intervention in breast oncology is not limited to medical aspects, but extends to facilitating the emotional balance and resilience of those affected. These professionals are prominent in guiding women to overcome the challenges imposed by the disease, favouring an environment of constant support. The ongoing support provided by nurses contributes to the efficient management of less visible symptoms, such as chronic fatigue and emotional distress, elements that are often underestimated in conventional therapies.

After the acute phase of treatment, the role of nurses in long-term surveillance persists, preventing relapses and monitoring adaptation to the necessary lifestyle changes. This care practice not only reinforces patients' safety and comfort, but also strengthens their autonomy and ability to manage their own health. The hypothesis is that the expansive and adaptive role of nurses in the MBC setting enriches the women's recovery trajectory, directly influencing their satisfaction and long-term therapeutic success. Investigating the effect of innovative nursing practices in this context is imperative to highlight the effectiveness of approaches that go beyond conventional treatment. Therefore, recognising these strategies can facilitate the implementation of more inclusive and comprehensive health policies that embrace the complexity of users' needs, culminating in a substantive improvement in standards of care in breast oncology. The relevance of innovative nursing methods applied to breast cancer treatment emphasises the urgency of moving beyond traditional medical devices. These modern techniques are fundamental to formulating more effective and inclusive health policies that correspond to the diversity of patients' needs, thus raising the standards of care in breast oncology. Within this context, the nurse stands out, whose role is indispensable from diagnosis to follow-up after treatment, offering care that addresses both the physical and emotional aspects of women. Investigating nurses' experiences provides an in-depth understanding of the interactions between the personal and professional spheres, bringing important perspectives for the development of better care practices.

Therefore, the adoption of a systematic review is indispensable to highlight nurse interventions and the need to associate these innovations in the management of pathology, providing an improvement in the properties of the treatment offered.

Therefore, by investigating nurses in the setting of breast cancer, it is possible to deepen our understanding of the qualifications and skills required to provide efficient care. In this way, the study analyses the nursing tactics used to mitigate the effects of the treatment, encouraging self-care and education for both patients and their families, providing emotional support throughout the process.

This study therefore addresses the following problem: How do nursing interventions influence the treatment and quality of life of breast cancer patients?

With this in mind, this study aims to carry out a systematic review of the impact of nursing actions on women with breast cancer.

2 OBJECTIVES

2.1 GENERAL OBJECTIVE

Carry out a systematic review on the impact of nursing actions on women with breast cancer.

2.2 SPECIFIC OBJECTIVES

- Identify the a actions performed by nursing in breast cancer prevention;
- To present the role of nurses in the recovery of patients affected by the pathology;
- Understanding care strategies for women with breast cancer.

3 THEORETICAL BACKGROUND

3.1 THE BREAST CANCER JOURNEY: FROM GENETICS TO THERAPY

Breast cancer can be caused by genetic, environmental and lifestyle factors, such as a family history of the disease, alcohol consumption and obesity. Although it is not possible to prevent breast cancer completely, early detection through mammography and regular self-exams increase the effectiveness of treatment and the chances of a cure (Rodrigues; Cruz; Paixão, 2015).

The issue of breast cancer is widely discussed at a global level, emphasising the importance of integrated strategies to tackle it. The variability in incidence rates between different regions implies the need for customised approaches that take into account the socio-cultural and economic peculiarities of each area. In developed countries, despite the availability of resources and advanced technology for detection and treatment, challenges persist in terms of standardising access to health services (Marinho, 2017).

Representing the second most common type of cancer, breast cancer has approximately 1.7 million new cases registered, which corresponds to around 25% of all malignant tumours in women. In addition, it was the fifth most lethal cause of cancer death, resulting in approximately 522,000 deaths in the general population in 2012. In the specific context of women, BC is the most prevalent type and has the highest mortality rate of all cancers in developing countries (Ferlay et al., 2015).

In the Latin American context, we face the reality of underdeveloped infrastructures and an unequal distribution of medical resources. This results in a proportion of cases being identified at advanced stages, where therapeutic options are more restricted and less effective. It is estimated that in Latin America, around 50 per cent of cancer cases are diagnosed in advanced stages, when there is no longer any possibility of a cure. In contrast, in Sweden, a developed nation, this proportion is less than 10 per cent of women diagnosed (Justo et al., 2017).

In Brazil, 59,700 new cases of breast cancer have been predicted for 2019, representing 29.5% of all malignant tumours in women, with an incidence rate of 56 cases per 100,000 inhabitants. In 2016, 16,069 women died from breast cancer, making it the leading cause of cancer mortality among Brazilian women (Silva et al., 2021).

As a result, approximately 40 per cent of breast cancer cases in the country are identified in advanced stages, specifically stages III and IV. The Northern Region has the highest incidence of these late diagnoses, reaching 42%, which negatively impacts the possibilities of effective treatment and compromises the favourable prognosis for patients. Evidence from international studies indicates that adopting measures for the early detection of cancer, when combined with appropriate treatment, contributes significantly to reducing mortality caused by the disease and increasing the chances of survival for affected women (Silva et al., 2021).

In this context, it is correct to say that breast cancer has both emotional and physical impacts. The suspicion of the disease triggers a series of emotions in women, including fear and a sense of loss, anguish, guilt, rejection and uncertainty about the future. It is common for patients to feel guilty after diagnosis, associating the disease with their lifestyle, lack of care for their bodies, the constant stress they are under and their genetic load. For these women, having breast cancer is often seen as synonymous with death and loss of self-image (Villar et al., 2017).

According to Marinho:

1) most cases of cancer are discovered by the woman herself; 2) MSA can lead to early detection between the period of clinical examination and mammography and 3) it may be the only method available to women who have difficulty getting an appointment with a qualified health professional or more sophisticated tests such as mammography (Marinho, 2017, p. 236).

The last two decades have seen remarkable progress in the processes of diagnosis and anti-cancer therapy, with updates and specifications in methods ranging from imaging to molecular biology techniques. These advances have enabled precise diagnoses, effective follow-up and accurate prognostic assessments for patients. Developments in both diagnostics and therapeutics have led to an increase in the survival of cases that were previously considered incurable (Nascimento; Pitta; Rego, 2015).

Most hereditary breast cancers are invasive tumours, with the infiltrating ductal type predominating, accounting for 65 to 80% of cases. Several factors influence the prognosis of the disease, such as axillary lymph node involvement, the main prognostic indicator, as well as tumour size and contour, histological type and grade, vascular invasion, presence of hormone receptors, tumour proliferation rates and the patient's age, with younger patients tending to have tumours with poorer prognoses (D'Ávila, 2016).

According to the explanation given by Arruda and his team, this is how cancer arises:

At the start of the mitotic cycle, the p53 gene transcriptionally activates the p21 gene, inducing the synthesis of the p21 protein, whose function is to inhibit the action of cyclin-dependent kinases (CDKs), causing the cell to stop in the G1 phase until it completes DNA repair. To do this, the p53 protein activates the GADD-45 gene (Growth Arrest DNA Damage Inducille), which acts to correct the DNA damage. If the lesion is extensive, p53 activates genes involved in the apoptosis mechanism, suppressing the action of genes with anti-apoptotic action (Arruda et al., 2018, p.126). Cancer treatment employs modalities such as surgery and radiotherapy for localised interventions, and chemotherapy and therapies with biological modulators for systemic approaches. The necessary treatments entail numerous detrimental changes to patients' quality of life (Nascimento; Pitta; Rego, 2015).

It should also be noted that delays in carrying out tests and the late start of treatment can significantly reduce the chances of cure and patient survival, as well as requiring more aggressive therapies, with the combined use of various therapeutic modalities and the consequent increase in sequelae and public costs due to more extensive and expensive treatments, as well as social security costs related to time off work (D'Ávila, 2016).

As for welcoming women with breast cancer, studies have highlighted its importance as a fundamental element in humanising healthcare. Through this welcome, nursing professionals show interest and willingness to establish bonds with patients and their families, addressing their care needs and alleviating fears related to the disease (Villar et al., 2017).

National campaigns, such as Pink October, help disseminate information about CM, reaching a wider audience. and promoting mass education. Training health professionals to deal empathetically and effectively with this issue is also an area that needs continuous improvement, aimed not only at appropriate treatment, but also at providing emotional support to patients (Rodrigues; Cruz; Paixão, 2015).

3.2 NURSES IN BREAST CANCER PREVENTION

Nurses play a crucial role in the fight against breast cancer, especially through preventive education and the promotion of a healthy lifestyle. These professionals are fundamental in disseminating knowledge about breast self-examination, enabling women to acquire the autonomy to carry out this practice, which is essential for the early detection of possible anomalies (Backes et al., 2019).

Through continuous instruction, this professional encourages the adoption of habits that are beneficial to health, such as maintaining a balanced diet, systematically practising physical activity and limiting alcohol consumption. These guidelines are vital as they directly contribute to reducing the risk of developing breast cancer and significantly improve women's quality of life (Dias et al., 2023).

In addition, nurses play a leading role in organising and implementing health education programmes. Using scientific methods, nurses actively empower women, enabling them to make informed decisions about their breast health. The nurse's leadership is decisive in providing qualified and humanised care, as supported by the following guidelines resolutions of the Federal Nursing Council (COFEN), such as numbers 358/2009, 210/1998 and 211/1998 (Mineo et al., 2015).

Cancer, often associated with feelings of fear, pain and suffering, requires a sensitive and empathetic approach from nurses. By recognising their own conceptions of the disease, nurses are called upon to develop coping strategies that minimise the suffering of those involved. Nursing care, when based on principles of empathy and understanding, becomes a fundamental component in supporting patients (Souza et al., 2020).With regard to oncology nurses: "The main focus is on controlling the adverse effects of treatment, assessing the demands made by the patient, monitoring the symptoms of the disease and the consequences of treatment on the patient's routine." (Souza et al., 2020, p.9)In this sense, the presence of nurses in primary health care is indispensable, since they act from prevention to support in the readaptation of patients after treatment. Through a comprehensive and continuous approach throughout the life cycle, nurses ensure health promotion and disease prevention, playing an irreplaceable role in the healthcare system. The interaction of these professionals with patients from the earliest stages is decisive for identifying risk factors and providing appropriate guidance on prevention practices and early detection of breast cancer (Rodrigues; Cruz; Paixão, 2015).

As such, nurses, as health educators and counsellors, are essential in transforming health scenarios, promoting not only the physical but also the emotional well-being of their patients. Their actions are based on scientific evidence and human sensitivity, always aiming for the best possible result in the healthcare process. breast cancer care and prevention journey (Dias et al., 2023; Souza et al., 2020).

3.3 NURSING AND THE DIAGNOSIS OF WOMEN WITH BREAST CANCER

The position of nursing in the hospital is the result of a combination of factors experienced in practice, which include the subjectivity of the professionals, the remnants of the history of the nursing profession, as well as others arising from organisational issues and the care and administrative models existing in healthcare establishments (Lunardi Filho, 2016).

According to Backes and scholars: "thinking about the professional practice of nurses involves, on the one hand, knowledge associated with social, economic and political macro-results, and, on the other, micro-spaces in which the nurse-patient and nurse-health professional relationship/interaction takes place." (Backes et al., 2016, p. 319). This guidance is essential to ensure that women understand the importance of imaging tests in the early detection of the disease and feel encouraged to undergo them regularly.

Another relevant aspect is the role of nursing in the psychosocial scenario of patients, that is, during the process of diagnosis of BC. As Garcia et al. point out, "nurses play an essential role in providing emotional support and accurate and understandable information to patients, helping to reduce the fear and anxiety associated with the diagnosis of the disease" (Garcia et al., 2020, p.115).

During the process of diagnosing breast neoplasia, nursing stands out when it comes to educating patients about the different stages of the pathology and the treatment options available. Thus, nurses emerge as an important figure in the prevention of breast cancer, as they advise women on self-examination and the importance of having a mammogram (Azevedo et al., 2017).

In addition to these responsibilities, nursing is involved in formulating strategies for managing women's health at various stages of life, emphasising the importance of regular monitoring and raising awareness about breast health. It plays a role in the diagnosis phase, as well as in monitoring users throughout the intervention, providing ongoing support and up-to-date information on treatment innovations (Backes et al., 2018).

Nursing practice in the context of CM also includes the implementation of community education programmes and awareness campaigns aimed at reaching a larger portion of the population. Such initiatives are designed to demystify the disease, promote knowledge about the symptoms and encourage women to seek timely medical attention (Lunardi Filho, 2016;

Backes et al., 2018).In light of this, through open dialogue and an empathetic approach, nurses help to build a relationship of trust with patients, which is fundamental to the success of treatments and the emotional well-being of those involved. They use their expertise to tailor information to the individual needs of each person, facilitating understanding and the active involvement of women in their care plans (Garcia et al., 2020). Nurses' work therefore reflects the intersection of technical skills with a strong human dimension, where sensitivity and commitment to the patient's dignity are just as important as diagnostic precision. This set of skillsand the comprehensive approach adopted by nurses are decisive in making progress in the fight against breast cancer and improving survival rates and quality of life for patients (Mineo et al., 2015).

3.4 NURSING AND THE MANAGEMENT OF BREAST CANCER PATIENT CARE

In the treatment of breast cancer, nursing stands out in the integrated management of care, going beyond medical interventions to embrace the coordination of services across the various levels of care. These professionals establish a relationship of trust and empathy with patients, which is fundamental for adherence and successful treatment. They are responsible for administering medication, monitoring adverse effects and offering emotional support, while also engaging in educational practices that motivate patients to become actively involved in their health process (Cunha, 2018).

At the same time, nurses encourage healthy lifestyle practices, which are essential for recovery and improving patients' quality of life. Guidance on a balanced diet, physical activity and stress management are integrated into care, with the aim of minimising the risk of the disease recurring. This multidimensional approach to nursing promotes patients' resilience, providing them with the tools they need to face the challenges of the disease and creating a care environment that is holistic and personalised (Azevedo et al., 2017).

According to Zinhani:

Nurses have a very important role to play in promoting health. health, as it promotes strategies and actions that can increase the quality of life of the population, as well as assisting in treatment more closely in the communities and, when necessary, carrying out home visits for those who need rehabilitation and palliative care, offering continuity of care in a comprehensive manner within the scope of primary health care (Zinhadi, 2018, p.86). Nurses are essential in the early detection of breast cancer, advising patients on the regularity of gynaecological appointments and the importance of diagnostic tests such as mammography. They encourage women to regularly monitor the condition of their breasts and to carry out self-examination when they feel comfortable. In addition, during consultations, prevention and health promotion initiatives are implemented, which are also covered in community talks for women (Nadal; Gonçalves, 2018). The nurse's contribution is also relevant, both in carrying out consultations and recommending fundamental tests, and in being involved in educational programmes, in which they act in prevention and help in the early diagnosis of the disease (Cunha, 2018). It is imperative that the multi-professional health team develops strategies focused on prevention and education about breast cancer and its treatments. These actions aim to provide knowledge to all those involved, enabling an organised approach to coping with the disease and offering the necessary support to patients and their families (Nadal; Gonçalves, 2018).To summarise, nurses have multiple responsibilities in the management of breast cancer treatment, ranging from the administration of therapies and symptom control to patient education and self-care support. Their comprehensive and dedicated work is fundamental to guaranteeing quality care at all stages of treatment. phases of treatment (Garcia et al., 2020).

3.5 NURSING'S CONTRIBUTIONS TO THE RECOVERY OF WOMEN WITH BREAST CANCER

Within breast cancer recovery, the participation of nurses is visible, as they fulfil a series of functions aimed at promoting the physical and emotional well-being of patients. These professionals have the autonomy to highlight crucial guidelines during nursing consultations, where they emphasise the importance of Clinical Breast Self-Examination (CBA), address normal and characteristic aspects of breast cancer and correctly perform the Clinical Breast Examination (CBE). In addition, nurses are responsible for listing actions to control the disease (Marins; Macedo; Vieira, 2017).

In this context, Wunder and scholars argue that:

The aim of the nursing consultation is to offer specialised, individualised care to the patient, using simple, easy-to-understand language, with the aim of providing guidance and clarification about the treatment, encouraging self-care, managing possible side effects, reviewing the symptomatic medication prescribed by the doctor, providing guidance on the importance of adequate hydration and nutrition, care to prevent infections and warning signs, thus favouring increased adherence and successful treatment. It is understood that the outpatient nursing consultation is an effective strategy, since it favours getting closer and building an interpersonal relationship of help, where the management of nursing care involves recognising and meeting the patient's care needs

(Wunder et al 2017, p. 28).In the field of care, nurses are responsible for creating strategies to prevent cancer through health education, working mainly in primary care. This role involves health promotion, prevention and protection, providing comprehensive care in a humanistic way (Souza et al., 2020).

In this sense, nursing practice in cancer should cover all age groups of women and integrate the basic knowledge of this area into all specialities, being carried out in any healthcare environment, from homes and communities to acute care institutions and rehabilitation centres (Recco; Luiz; Pinto, 2020). It is important to emphasise that nursing care is provided by a team made up of nurses, technicians and nursing assistants, whose duties are outlined by Decree 94.406/87, making nurses responsible for drawing up, implementing and evaluating health care plans, with a view to preventing and controlling possible damage to the patient's health (Stumm et al., (2018). In addition, it is essential for nurses to advise patients to carry out breast self-examination periodically, between 7 and 10 days after the start of menstruation. For women who no longer menstruate, who are in the menopause, who have had their uterus removed or who are breastfeeding, it is crucial to provide guidance on choosing a day each month to carry out the self-examination (Rodrigues et al., 2019).The inclusion of the nursing team in the care of cancer patients requires clear knowledge, skills and responsibilities aimed at the patient, their family and other significant people, taking into account the physical, emotional, social and spiritual aspects (Stumm et al., (2018). According to Lima and Machado: When a woman receives a diagnosis of breast cancer and information about the disease and treatment, she is faced with the fragility of her existence and the possibility of death becomes present in her thoughts. This he diagnosis brings many changes to the patient's life and routine, as it generates a great deal of emotional conflict, going through stages ranging from denial to acceptance of the diagnosis, since cancer is still seen as an incurable disease. The psychological state, not only of the patient, but also of the whole family becomes vulnerable, with a predominant feeling of fear at the unexpected experience they will go through (Lima; Machado, 2018, p. 88). It is therefore extremely important for nurses to take part in multidisciplinary actions, from prevention to diagnosis and recovery, since encompassing educational proposals favours greater knowledge on the subject. To this end, nurses must be trained to understand attitudes and fears when planning actions to improve the quality of life of these patients (Cavalcante et al., 2016).

Therefore, nurses can also order complementary tests for investigation based on inter-municipal administrative protocols, give talks and make community visits, promoting guidance on risk factors for breast cancer (Sales, 2017).

4 METHODOLOGY

This is a systematic review of the impact of nursing actions on women with breast cancer. The research was based on a broad scan of the literature, using recognised databases such as MEDLINE (Medical Literature Analysis and Retrieval System Online), LILACS (Latin American and Caribbean Health Sciences Literature) and BDENF (Nursing Database).

The search strategy used the BVS (Virtual Health Library) portal to access the databases mentioned. The descriptors were selected using DeCS (Health Sciences Descriptors) and MeSH (Medical Subject Headings), choosing terms such as "Nursing Care", "Breast Neoplasms" and "Oncology". The terms were combined in the databases using the Boolean operators "AND" and "OR".

The research followed the standards set by the PRISMA statement, including a 27-item checklist and a flow chart to structure the review in a clear and systematic way (Moher et al.,2009; Urrútia; Bonfill, 2010).

Articles were selected between February and May 2024. An initial survey of 300 studies was carried out, with the following distribution: 150 in MEDLINE, 90 in LILACS and 60 in BDENF. After applying preliminary filters with the availability of full text, language (Portuguese) and publications between 2019 and 2024, 200 studies were discarded in order to answer the problem: How do nursing interventions influence the treatment and quality of life of breast cancer patients?

Following this procedure, 60 of the remaining 100 articles were removed for duplication. After reviewing the title and abstract, 25 studies were excluded because they did not fully meet the thematic relevance criteria, leaving 15 articles for eligibility assessment. Of these, 5 were discarded after a detailed evaluation, culminating in the selection of 10 studies for full analysis.However, the inclusion criteria covered original articles, published in the last five years and in Portuguese, which explicitly detailed nursing interventions for women with breast cancer. Therefore, studies without full access, publications prior to 2019, repeated works and those that, after careful reading of the abstracts and full texts, did not meet the objectives of this review were excluded.

Therefore, the analysis of the data collected was systematised using a table that recorded the author(s), year of publication, title of the work, database used, sample and main results. The interpretation and critical analysis of the data was carried out comparatively, with the aim of drawing conclusions about the impact of nursing practices on the treatment and recovery of breast cancer patients.

See the diagram below:

Figure 1 - Process flow for selecting scientific articles

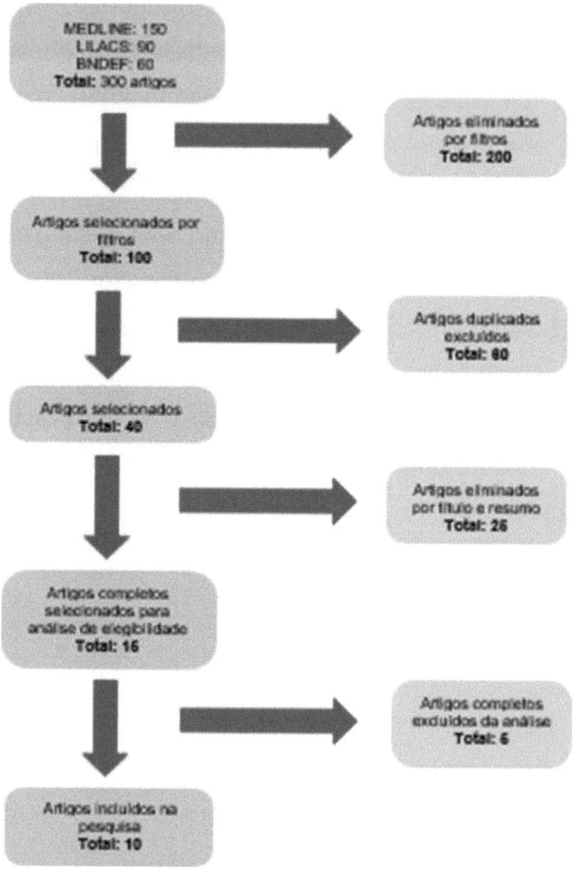

MEDLINE: 150
LILACS: 90
BNDEF: 60
Total: 300 artigos

Artigos eliminados por filtros
Total: 200

Artigos selecionados por filtros
Total: 100

Artigos duplicados excluídos
Total: 60

Artigos selecionados
Total: 40

Artigos eliminados por título e resumo
Total: 26

Artigos completos selecionados para análise de elegibilidade
Total: 16

Artigos completos excluídos da análise
Total: 6

Artigos incluídos na pesquisa
Total: 10

Source: Author

5 RESULTS AND DISCUSSIONS

The systematic review carried out contributes significantly to deepening the understanding of the anatomo-physiological complexity of breast cancer, highlighting its critical importance for both oncology and other medical areas. This depth of knowledge is essential in clinical practice, as it provides a detailed overview of the biological structures involved and their implications for tumour development and progression.

The detailed study selected data from recent and relevant scientific research that elucidates the multiple facets of breast cancer. This research helps to clarify the individual variations and patterns of manifestation of the disease, favouring a better understanding of its peculiarities and complexities. Integrating this new data with the existing literature is fundamental to ensuring a holistic and up-to-date understanding, allowing for advances in the treatment and management of the pathology.

However, as well as compiling and analysing the data, the review also highlighted the importance of measures in the treatment of breast cancer. Collaboration between oncologists, radiologists, surgeons, nurses and other healthcare professionals is essential to develop an effective treatment plan that addresses all aspects of the disease. This integrated approach improves clinical outcomes and tends to better support patients throughout the entire care process, from diagnosis to recovery and long-term follow-up.

The results also reinforce the need for ongoing research to explore new therapies and treatment strategies. With the advance of technologies and the evolution of medical techniques, therefore, new opportunities are constantly arising for optimise patients' quality of life and increase survival rates. It is therefore vital that the scientific community maintains a constant commitment to updating and deepening knowledge in the field. In order to systematise and clearly present the results obtained, a table will follow this discussion. Called Table 1, it not only facilitates access to the information collected, but also enables a comparative analysis with the data already established in the scientific corpus. This element is essential to highlight the contributions of each selected study to the global understanding of breast cancer, underlining the importance and impact of each piece of data analysed in understanding the disease. See table 1 below:

Table 1 - Articles used in the systematic review

No. Order	Author/Year	Title	Type of study/Sample	Relevant results
1	Melo et al. (2023)	Nursing diagnoses based on the repercussions of breast cancer and mastectomy	Descriptive, qualitative research carried out at an NGO in João Pessoa, PB. Sample of 15 mastectomised women between September and October 2017. Semi-structured interviews Analysed analysed using Bardin's Content Analysis Technique.	Nursing diagnoses were identified based on three thematic categories: feelings after diagnosis and mastectomy; biological and psychological changes after mastectomy; and resilience in the face of suffering. Socio-economic data indicates that 33.4 per cent of the women are aged 56-62, 40 per cent are widows, 40 per cent have primary education, 80 per cent are Catholic, and 53.4 per cent have an income of up to one minimum wage. Diagnoses include distress, Impaired well-being, altered self-esteem and self-image, among others.
2	Andreazzi et al. (2022)	The role of nursing with mastectomised women: aspects sentimental	Qualitative, descriptive literature review. Data collection in the Virtual Health Library, analysis of 10 articles from December 2016 to December 2021. Bardin Content Analysis used.	Women who have been diagnosed with breast cancer and have undergone mastectomy often experience negative feelings such as fear, insecurity, low self-esteem, feelings of abandonment, depression, reduced sexuality and sadness. The work of the nursing team is crucial, providing support and comfort, making it possible to reduce these negative feelings. No specific percentages of the results were presented.

Continued from Table 1 - Articles used in the systematic review

No. Order		Author/ Year	Title	Type of study/Sample	Relevant results
3		Moura et al. (2022)	Nurses' perceptions of nurses about early detection and prevention of breast cancer in primary health care primary health care	A descriptive, qualitative study, carried out in Basic Health Units in a city in the interior of São Paulo with 12 nurses.	All the nurses demonstrated knowledge of their responsibilities in preventive strategies for the early detection of breast cancer. The COVID-19 pandemic has negatively affected the implementation of preventive strategies due to social distancing and the population's fear of seeking health services. The nurses reported practical difficulties due to work overload, with 50% of the nurses being single and 75% having a specialisation, indicating a profile of a highly qualified but pressured team.100% of the participants are female.100 per cent of the participants were female, aged between 27 and 36, highlighting a young and predominantly female group in the organisation. front line.
4		Oliveira et al. (2021)	Caring for people with metastatic breast cancer in primary care	Qualitative research, case report. Data collected in May 2019 through two home visits and family family medical records.	The care defined included: encouraging hydration, controlling nausea and vomiting, and improving tissue integrity. The importance of implementing the nursing process was highlighted for the systematisation of shared care, favouring comprehensive and longitudinal care, as well as the family

					focus of primary care actions.
5		Souza et al. (2021)	Itineraries treatment of women with breast cancer: perceptions of primary health care nurses	Exploratory, descriptive study approach qualitative, carried out with 8 nurses working in the Family Health Strategy in a municipality in Santa Catarina. Data collected through interviews semi-structured interviews in the second half of 2018.	The nurses identified the offer of free treatment by the SUS and the municipality's status as a reference for oncological treatment as advantages. Difficulties included the lack of protocols to increase nurses' autonomy and the inefficiency of referral and counter-referral flows. The need for ongoing education and the establishment of clear flows to improve care and reduce the incidence of cancer was emphasised. of the disease.

Continued from Table 1 - Articles used in the systematic review

No. Order		Author/ Year	Title	Type of study/Sample	Relevant results
6		Merênc io and Ventur a (2020)	Women's experiences mastectomy: rehabilitatio n nursing to promote autonomy	A phenomenolo gical qualitative study. Sample of 9 women mastectomise d interviewed in their homes using the snowball method.	Difficulties in home adaptation included persistent pain and limitations in arm mobility on the mastectomy side, with some women developing lymphoedema, estimated at 20-25% of women undergoing surgery. Fear, sadness and anger were common feelings, with a significant impact on body image and interpersonal relationships. Rehabilitation was essential for regaining functionality and accepting the new body image, but less than 25 per cent of women received adequate home rehabilitation.
7		Reis et al. (2019)	Confrontatio n of women who have experienced breast cancer	Qualitative study, interviews with 13 womenunderg oing chemotherapy .	38% of the participants were under the age of 50, 23% were in stage III cancer, and 54% had their left breast affected. The study identified that coping with cancer occurs at all stages of the disease, as a way of overcoming the difficulties of the disease. treatments and social impacts.

8		Pereira (2020)	Manual educational programme for women with breast cancer undergoing chemotherapy	Qualitative study usingResearch Convergent Assistance (PCA). Data collected Through of interviews semi-structured with 16 women treated at a public hospital in southern Brazil.	There was a range between 35 and 59 years of age, with 44 per cent of women in the 40-49 age group. 37.5 per cent of the women were in stage II breast cancer, while 25 per cent were in stages I and III respectively. Around 30 per cent of the participants expressed concerns about their self-image and self-esteem due to the effects of chemotherapy. However, strategies for managing side effects, such as nausea and hair loss, were discussed and were useful for approxImately 75% of the participants. of the interviewees.

The study carried out by Melo and his colleagues highlights the complexity of nursing diagnoses in mastectomised women, identifying three main thematic categories: emotional reactions to the diagnosis and surgery, subsequent biological and psychological changes, and the patients' capacity for resilience. This research also shows socio-economic data, highlighting the distribution of age, marital status, level of education, religion and income, which helps to understand the context in which these women are inserted. Andreazzi et al. (2022) carried out a meticulous review of the literature focusing on how patients face the emotional challenges associated with breast cancer and mastectomy. This research highlights the relevance of nursing practice, emphasising its ability to provide both emotional and practical support in extremely complex moments. The results show that feelings of fear, insecurity and depression are prevalent, but can be mitigated through carefully designed and executed nursing interventions.

Furthermore, both studies analysed reiterate the critical importance of the nurse's role in reducing the adverse emotional impacts resulting from the diagnosis and treatment of BC. There is no disagreement between the conclusions of these studies, but they present different perspectives on strategies to manage the complex demands faced by women. This illustrates the need for an adaptive practice that fully considers the physical and emotional aspects involved in recovery and strengthening the well-being of those involved.

Consequently, the synergy between these studies strengthens the understanding that integrated management that is sensitive to the particularities of each patient is essential for effective care. Therefore, this expanded approach suggests that nursing practices must continually evolve in order to effectively and empathetically meet the varied needs during the rehabilitation process, ensuring that the intervention is both inclusive and comprehensive.

In the study carried out by Merêncio and Ventura (2020), the investigation into the experiences of mastectomised women offers significant depth and complements the findings of previous research, such as those by Melo et al. (2023) and Andreazzi et al. (2022). The focus of this additional article on the rehabilitation process and the promotion of female autonomy post-mastectomy emphasises the importance of practices that strengthen emotional support and physical independence, as well as patients' self-image.

In detail, Merêncio and Ventura (2020) emphasise that nursing intervention in the rehabilitation process can play an important role in facilitating a more integrated recovery. This type of care encompasses both the physical and psychological needs of patients, establishing a parallel with the findings of Melo et al. (2023), who emphasise the resilience and support needed to adapt to biological and psychological changes. Thus, the analysis by Andreazzi et al. (2022) distinguishes how the impact of negative feelings can be mitigated when there is effective nursing action, providing comfort and emotional support.

Merêncio and Ventura's (2020) contribution to the field of study offers a more comprehensive view, highlighting the need for nursing services that alleviate the adverse emotional aspects associated with breast cancer and mastectomy. Such care should promote physical recovery as well as women's autonomy.

These studies collectively reinforce the view that the recovery of mastectomised women transcends the physical dimension, engaging also in the emotional and psychological spheres. However, this integrated approach suggests that nursing interventions must be carefully planned to address the multiple aspects of patients' lives, which can include everything from the administration of physical therapies to psychological and emotional support. According to the publication by Moura et al. (2022), it brings a new dimension to the understanding of the challenges faced by women with breast cancer, by focussing solely on early detection strategies and prevention adopted in primary health care. According to Moura et al, early and educational interventions can positively influence the health management of these patients, favouring the reduction and incidence of the severity of CM through effective surveillance and health education.

Moura et al. (2022) also examined the effectiveness of nursing practices in advising women on the importance of regular examinations and raising awareness of the risk factors associated with BC. This preventive approach is essential, as early detection is important for improving prognosis and reducing mortality rates related to the disease.

In addition, the research by Douberin et al. (2019) tends to deepen knowledge about the treatment of women with breast cancer, focusing on the comorbidities that often coexist with the disease. The research reveals a prevalence of conditions such as hypertension and diabetes among these patients, highlighting the clinical management needed to optimise therapeutic results.

By elucidating the occurrence of multiple diseases, the research by Douberin et al. (2019) emphasises the need for an adapted therapeutic tactic that analyses breast cancer and the various comorbidities that can affect the effectiveness of the procedure and the restoration of patients. This approach is substantial for drawing up personalised care plans that focus on improving the quality of life of these women.

Given this, the work of Douberin and his team complements the studies by Moura et al. (2022), reinforcing the importance of comprehensive action in cancer care. However, the differences are not explicit, but can be inferred from the different emphasis of each study, such as those that focus more on practical and clinical aspects (Douberin et al., 2019; Moura et al., 2022) versus those that focus on subjective and emotional experiences (Melo et al., 2023; Merêncio; Ventura, 2020).

In contrast, the works by Oliveira, Isidoro and Silva (2021) and Souza et al. (2021) bring strong reinforcements and additions to the literature on oncological care, explaining different points of care for patients with neoplasms.

The study by Oliveira, Isidoro and Silva (2021) focuses on the implementation of cancer care in primary care, especially in cases of metastasis. The authors highlight the success of a home care model that allows for continuity and personalisation of treatment, stressing the importance of adapting care to individual needs, i.e. managing symptoms within the family.

On the other hand, Souza et al. (2021) investigated the conceptions of women with breast cancer about nursing care, focusing on the spiritual dimension of treatment. The publication points out that patients highly value the sensitivity and understanding of nurses in relation to their emotional and spiritual challenges, pointing to the need for a method that integrates psychological and spiritual support as a fundamental part of neoplastic treatment.

From a similar angle, Reis, Panobianco and Gradim (2019) show the dynamics of coping in women who have experienced BC, exploring the nuances of the treatment process and the interaction of these patients with the healthcare system. The authors used a qualitative methodology to deepen their understanding of how these people cope with the diagnosis and subsequent oncological intervention, emphasising the importance of appropriate psychological support. The analysis revealed that effective coping is relevant to women's adaptation to the various stages of treatment, from diagnosis to recovery, and that this process is significantly influenced by the quality of communication and relationships with health professionals.

The results indicate that a high proportion of women find the healthcare team, especially the nurses, to be a pillar of emotional support. This support is seen as a mitigating factor against the emotional repercussions of breast cancer. Among the variables that directly affect coping, the clarity of the information provided, the empathy of health professionals and the availability of therapeutic resources stand out. These elements are fundamental to strengthening users' ability to cope with the disease, explicitly stimulating their well-being.

Pereira (2020) focuses on the development and application of an educational manual for women undergoing chemotherapy for BC. Pereira's research used the Convergent Care Research (CCR) methodology, actively engaging patients in the process of developing the material. However, this manual was designed to provide information about the pathology, chemotherapy side effects, self-care strategies and symptom management techniques.

Including patients in the development of the educational material not only ensured that the content was relevant and tailored to their experiences, but also gave the women a sense of autonomy and control over their own treatment. The manual proved to be a tool for optimising patients' understanding of the disease and therapy, contributing to greater adherence to the prescribed interventions and better management of effects This has resulted in a remarkable improvement in the quality of life of the patients involved.

Although both articles focus on different aspects of the breast cancer experience, they emphasise the need for approaches that consider the individual as a whole. Reis, Panobianco and Gradim (2019) highlight the importance of emotional support in the coping process, while Pereira emphasises the need for information and education as forms of empowerment.The combination of these studies reinforces the idea that the effectiveness of treatment for BC is not limited to biomedical interventions; it is also intrinsically linked to the psychological, educational and emotional support offered to patients. This perspective is fundamental to promoting the health and well-being of women facing this challenging condition. Sequentially, the research by Birk et al. (2019) presents an in-depth analysis of the perceptions of women with MBC regarding the spiritual care offered during treatment. The study, set in the context of a specialised hospital, involved a series of in-depth interviews with patients going through different stages of cancer treatment, including chemotherapy and radiotherapy. The researchers sought to understand how spiritual care, when integrated with conventional treatments, can influence the well-being and recovery of people undergoing oncological procedures.

Birk et al.'s (2019) approach to spirituality in the clinical context addresses a dimension that is often neglected in oncology. Spirituality, as identified by the study, is an aspect of the human experience, notably for patients facing serious and life-threatening illnesses such as breast cancer. The study revealed that the majority of patients highly valued

o spiritual support as part of their care plan, as it provides comfort, hope and a sense of purpose amidst the adversity of illness.

The methodology adopted by the researchers was semi-structured interviews, which allowed the participants to freely express their experiences and feelings related to cancer and the treatment they had received. The data collected was analysed using the content analysis technique, which facilitated the identification of recurring themes in the patients' narratives. These themes included the importance of the human and empathetic presence of healthcare professionals, the value of prayer and meditation, and the positive impact of spiritual support on coping with pathology. One of the most important findings of the study was the correlation between spiritual support and patients' resilience. Many reported that faith and spiritual practices were fundamental elements in maintaining a positive attitude during treatment. Furthermore, integrating spirituality into care proved to be beneficial not only for the patients, but also for strengthening the relationship between them and the healthcare team, promoting a more holistic, woman-centred approach.

The practical implications of their writings recommend that hospitals and cancer treatment centres should consider applying structured spiritual care programmes, which could include interventions for nurses and doctors on how to address spiritual issues sensitively. In addition, the study pointed to the need to create physical spaces in hospitals that promote tranquillity and recollection, such as chapels or gardens, where patients and families can find peace and comfort. In this way, the article by Birk et al. (2019) makes a valuable contribution to the field of oncology, offering evidence that spiritual care is an important dimension in the treatment of BC. By highlighting how this type of care can improve patients' well-being, the publication challenges healthcare professionals to rethink their practices and adopt a more inclusive and compassionate vision of therapeutic actions. Ratifying the idea of treating the patient as a whole, recognising and meeting people's physical, emotional and spiritual requirements, ensuring a cohesive and respected method.

In light of the above, the extensive literature points to the importance of incorporating educational factors, as well as psychological and spiritual support, corroborating the need for comprehensive care that accompanies women in all aspects of their journey. However, these investigations propose a clinical practice that values the whole person, promoting not only physical recovery, but also emotional invigoration and health progress, both during and after anti-cancer therapy.

6 CONCLUSION

This study provided a detailed and comprehensive analysis of the influence of nursing interventions on breast cancer treatment and patients' quality of life. The research focused specifically on elucidating how these interventions shape the course of treatment and affect patients' well-being, achieving an in-depth understanding of the dynamics involved in this process. Answering the question, "How do nursing interventions influence the treatment and quality of life of breast cancer patients?", the systematised research revealed significant results. Through the systematic review, the objectives outlined were fully achieved. Firstly, nursing actions in breast cancer prevention were highlighted, with a special focus on health education and promoting self-care. These practices proved crucial not only for prevention, but also for early detection of the disease, which is fundamental for improving patients' prognoses. Awareness-raising and the adoption of preventive measures are essential in reducing the incidence of breast cancer.

Secondly, the study examined the role of nurses in the recovery period of patients, highlighting the importance of continuous and personalised care. By tailoring their care to the specific needs of each patient, nurses facilitate adaptation to physical and emotional changes, providing a smoother transition to resuming daily activities. This continuous support, which covers both physical and emotional aspects, is vital for effective recovery. In addition, the care strategies implemented by nurses to manage side effects and provide emotional support during treatment were identified and analysed. These strategies are fundamental to improving patients' quality of life, showing that the nursing approach goes beyond medical treatment to an integrative and humanised practice that considers the patient as a whole.

Continued from Table 1 - Articles used in the systematic review

No. Order		Author/ Year	Title	Type of study/Sample	Relevant results
9		Douberin et al. (2019)	Main comorbidities associated neoplasm breast under treatment chemotherapy	A quantitative, descriptive cross-sectional study of 317 women in a public hospital.	Of the 317 women studied, 115 (36,3%) reported comorbidities. Systemic arterial hypertension was the most prevalent, affecting 75 of the women with comorbidities (65.2% of 115). Diabetes mellitus was reported by 42 women (36.5% of 115). In addition In addition, 79 women (68.7 per cent of 115) had other conditions, including obesity. Around 7 per cent of the participants also reported facing depression.
10		Birk et al. (2019)	Perception of women with breast cancer on nursing care for spirituality	A qualitative, descriptive study carried out in 2015 with 14 women undergoing treatment chemotherapy for breast cancer in a teaching hospital .	Ages ranged from 30 to 70. 50 per cent of the women were between stages II and III of the cancer, and the remaining 28.6 per cent were in stage IV. The majority, 78.6%, had completed high school or higher education. They all lived in urban areas, 50% were married, and only one had no children.

Source: Author (2024)

The publication by Melo et al. (2023) and Andreazzi et al. (2022) present complementary perspectives on the impact of breast cancer and mastectomy on patients. Both papers focus on the constitutional role of nursing in managing the emotional and physical consequences of these medical circumstances.

The results emphasise the importance of continuing education and institutional support as foundations for the evolution of nursing practices, highlighting the need for health policies that promote continuous professional development and innovation in health care. With this, the research reiterates the need for new studies that can further explore the dimensions of nursing practices, with the aim of continually improving therapeutic and support approaches.

It is therefore concluded that the study successfully achieved its objectives, providing information for the field of oncology nursing and highlighting the urgent need for advances in health policies that effectively recognise and integrate the transformative role of nursing in breast cancer care. In this way, this study not only confirms the positive impact of nursing interventions in improving clinical outcomes, but also in promoting a more rewarding and humanised treatment experience for women with breast cancer.

REFERENCES

ANDREAZZI, A. L. P.; LAHAN, D. C. R.; FACIOLI, N. C. L.; SILVA, T. G.; BATISTA,

M. A.; LEAL, C. C. G. Nursing work with mastectomised women: sentimental aspects. **Cuid Enferm.**, v. 16, n. 1, p. 128-134, jan.-jun. 2022. Available in: https://docs.fundacaopadrealbino.com.br/media/documentos/c6d9443151 3ee776b23 6d29ed7bf7f46.pdf. Accessed on: 7 August 2024.

ARRUDA, J. T.; BORDIN, B. M.; MIRANDA, L. C. B.; MAIA, D. L. M.; MOURA, K. K.V. de O. P53 Protein and Cancer: Controversies and Hopes. **Estudos**, Goiânia, v. 35, p. 123-141, jan/feb 2018.

AZEVEDO, M. E. C.; ARAÚJO, C. C. de; CAMPOS, K. S.; RODRIGUES, R. P. de M.;SILVA, F. M. C. da. The role of nurses in breast cancer prevention: an integrative review. In: **CONBRACIS, II., 2017, Campina Grande**. Proceedings. Campina Grande: Realise Editora, 2017. Available at   at: https://editorarealize.com.br/artigo/visualizar/29110. Accessed on: 20 July 2024.

BACKES, D. S.; BACKES, M. S.; ERDMANN, A. L.; BÜSCHER, A. O papel profissional

of nurses in the Unified Health System: from community health to the family health strategy. **Ciência & Saúde Coletiva**, v. 17, n. 1, p. 223-230, jan. 2019. Available in: https://www.scielo.br/j/csc/a/B4YNT5WFyKmn5GNGbYBhCsD/?lang=pt&format=pdf. Accessed on: 27 July 2024.

BACKES, D. S.; BACKES, M. S.; SOUSA, F. G. M. de.; ERDMANN, A. L O papel do nurse in the hospital context: the vision of health professionals. **Cienc cuid saúde**, v. 7, n. 3, p. 319-26, 2016. Available at:

https://www.periodicos.uem.br/ojs/index.php/CiencCuidSaude/article/view/ 6490/3857. Accessed on: 27 July 2024.

BIRK, N. M.; GIRARDON-PERLINI, N. M. O.; LACERDA, M. R.; TERRA, M. G.;BEUTER, M.; MARTINS, F. C. Feelings experienced by women infected with HPV upon learning of the diagnosis of the disease. **Cienc Cuid Saude**, v. 18, n. 1, e45504, jan.-mar. 2019.

CAVALCANTE, S.A.M.; SILVA, F.B.; MARQUES, C.A.V.; FIGUEIREDO, E.N.F.;GUTIÉRREZ, M.G.R. Nurse actions in breast cancer screening and diagnosis in Brazil. **Revista Brasileira de Cancerologia**. v. 59, n. 3, p. 459-466, 2016.

CUNHA, A. R. The role of nurses in the guidance, promotion and prevention of breast cancer. **Revista Humano Ser - UNIFACEX**, v. 3, n. 1, p. 160-173, 2018.

D'AVILA, K. G. **Breast cancer**. Porto Alegre: Federal Faculty of Medical Sciences of Porto Alegre Foundation, 2016.

DIAS, L.; CALVI, A.; SIQUEIRA, D. DA S.; BORGHETTI, M. M. O papel do enfermeiro on the prevention and control of hospital-acquired infections in a care unit adult intensive care. **Revista de Saúde Dom Alberto**, v. 10, n. 1, p. 45-68, 2023. Available in:

https://revista.domalberto.edu.br/revistadesaudedomalberto/article/view/8 11/733. Accessed on: 30 July 2024.

DOUBERIN, C. A.; SILVA, L. S. R. da; MATOS, D. P. et al. Main comorbidities associated with breast neoplasia in chemotherapy treatment. **Rev. enferm. UFPE online**, Recife, v. 13, n. 5, p. 1295-1299, May 2019. Available at:

https://periodicos.ufpe.br/revistas/revistaenfermagem/article/view/238540/ 32230.Accessed on: 9 August 2024.

FERLAY, J.; SOERJOMATARAM, I.; DIKSHIT, R.; ESER, S.;

MATHERS, C.;REBELO, M. Cancer incidence and mortality worldwide: Sources, methods and major patterns in Globocan 2012. **International Journal of Cancer**, v. 136, n. 5, p. E359- E86, 2015.

GARCIA, A. L.; PEREIRA, M. G.; RODRIGUES, J. The role of nurses in the early diagnosis of breast cancer. **Revista de Pesquisa em Enfermagem**, v. 18, n. 2, p. 115-122, 2020.

JUSTO, N.; WILKING, N.; JÖNSSON, B.; LUCIANI, S.; CAZAP, E. Review of the treatment and outcomes of breast cancer in Latin America. **Oncologist**, v. 18,n. 3,p.248-256,2013. Available at: https://academic.oup.com/oncolo/article/18/3/248/6410202?login=false. Accessed on: 27 July 2024.

LIMA, C.P.; MACHADO, M.A. Main carers facing the experience of death: their senses and meanings. **Psicologia: Ciência e Profissão**, v. 38, n. 1, p. 88-102, 2018. Available in: https://www.scielo.br/j/pcp/a/DLfY9CJN9H9gsS5kBr7TPsv/?lang=pt&format=pdf. Accessed on: 27 July 2024.

LUNARDI FILHO, W. D. **The myth of the subordination of nursing work to medicine.** Pelotas: Editora e Gráfica Universitária - UFPel, 2016.

MARINS, G et al. The role of nurses in the early detection of breast cancer. **Electronic scientific journal of applied sciences from FAIT**, Itapeva, 17 Jan 2017,p. 1-10.

MARINHO, L. A. B. The role of breast self-examination and mammography in the early diagnosis of breast cancer. **Rev. ciênc. méd.**, (Campinas), Campinas, v. 11, n. 3, p. 233-242, Sept./Dec.,2017. Available in: http://biblioteca.ricesu.com.br/ler.php?art_cod=1274. Accessed on: 28 July 2024.

MELO, A. C.; ANDRADE, S. S.; MATOS, S. D.; GOMES, A. C.;

CERQUEIRA, A. C.;

VIEIRA, K. F.; LUCENA, A. L. R. Nursing diagnoses based on the repercussions of breast cancer and mastectomy. **Enferm Foco,** v. 14, e-202317, 2023. Disponível em: https://doi.org/10.21675/2357-707X.2023.v14.e-202317. Accessed on: 5 August 2024.

MERÊNCIO, K. M.; VENTURA, M. C. A. Experiences of mastectomised women: rehabilitation nursing in promoting autonomy. **Revista de Enfermagem Referência**, Série V, n.º 2, e19082, 2020. Available: https://scielo.pt/pdf/ref/vserVn2/vserVn2a13.pdf. Accessed on: 9 August 2024.

MINEO, F. L. V. et al. Nursing care in breast cancer treatment. **Revista Gestão & Saúde**, v. 4, n. 2, p. 2238-2260, 2015.

MOURA, T. S.; MAGALHÃES, P. A. P. de; FELTRIN, A. F. dos S.; SILVA, T. A. da.

Nurses' perception of early detection and prevention of breast cancer in primary health care. **Cuid Enferm.**, v. 16, n. 1, p. 93-100, jan.-jun. 2022. Disponível em: https://doi.org/10.21675/2357-707X.2023.v14.e-202317. Accessed on: 8 Aug. 2024.

MOHER, D., LIBERATI, A., TETZLAFF, J., ALTMAN, D.G., & PRISMA Group. Preferred reporting items for systematic reviews and meta-analyses: the PRISMA statement. **PLoS Medicine**, v.6, n.7, e1000097, 2009.

NASCIMENTO, F. B.; PITTA, M. G. R.; RÊGO, M. J. B. M. Analysis of the main breast cancer diagnosis methods as drivers in the innovation process. **Revista Arquivos de Medicina**, Porto, v. 29, n. 6, p. 153-159, 2015.

NADAL, B. S.; GONÇALVES, B. S. J. role of nurses in breast cancer prevention in primary care. Uniatenas, 2018.

OLIVEIRA, P. E.; ISIDORO, G. M.; SILVA, S. A. Caring for people with metastatic breast cancer in primary care: a case report. **J. Nurs. Health**, v. 11, n. 2, e2111219232,2021.Availableat: https://periodicos.ufpel.edu.br/ojs2/index.php/enfermagem/article/view/192 32. Accessed on: 8 Aug. 2024.

PEREIRA, S. C. da C. Educational manual for women with breast cancer undergoing chemotherapy. Dissertation (Master's in Healthcare Practice) **- Health Sciences Sector**, Federal University of Paraná, Curitiba, 2020. Available at: https://acervodigital.ufpr.br/xmlui/bitstream/handle/1884/70028/R%20- %20D%20%20SANELE%20CRISTINA%20DA%20CRUZ%20PEREIRA.p df?sequence=1&isAllowed=y. Accessed on: 8 August 2024.

RECCO, D. C.; LUIZ, C. B.; PINTO, M. H. The care provided to patients with cancer: from the point of view of a group of nurses from a large hospital in the interior of the state of São Paulo. **Health Science Archive**. São Paulo, 2020.

REIS, A. P. A.; PANOBIANCO, M. S.; GRADIM, C. V. C. Coping of women who have experienced breast cancer. **Revista de Enfermagem do Centro-Oeste Mineiro**,v. 9,e2758, 2019.Availableat: https://seer.ufsj.edu.br/recom/article/view/2758/2079. Accessed on: 5 August 2024.

RODRIGUES, F. B.; ALMEIDA, A. A.; FONTINELE, D. C. S. S.; SILVEIRA JÚNIOR, L. S.; OLIVEIRA, S. P. S.; PAULINO, T. S. C. O papel do enfermeiro na prevenção do breast cancer in a municipality in the Pernambuco hinterland: an approach to professional practice. **Saúde Coletiva Debate**, 2019, v. 2, n. 1, p. 73-86.

RODRIGUES, J. D.; CRUZ, M. S.; PAIXÃO, A. N. An analysis of breast cancer prevention in Brazil. **Journal Ciência & Saúde Coletiva**, Rio de Janeiro, v. 20,

n. 10, p. 3163- 76, 2015.

SALES, M. A. Ductal carcinoma in situ of the breast: criteria for diagnosis and approach in public hospitals in Belo Horizonte. **Revista Brasileira de Ginecologia e obstetrícia**, Rio de Janeiro, v. 28, n°12, dezembro, 2017.

SILVA, M. S. B.; GUTIÉRREZ, M. G. R.; FIGUEIREDO, E. N.; BARBIERI, M.; RAMOS,
C. F. V.; GABRIELLONI, M. C. Actions for the early detection of breast cancer in two municipalities in the Western Amazon. **Revista Brasileira de Enfermagem**, v. 74, n.2,e20200165, 2021.Available at: https://www.scielo.br/j/reben/a/NSp4QQQvY7XJ5cYBNmjNNFS/?format= pdf&lang=pt. Accessed on: 30 July 2024.
SOUZA, J. B.; MANOROV, M.; MARTINS, E. L.; REIS, L.; BUSS HEIDEMANN, I. T.
S. Therapeutic itineraries of women with breast cancer: perceptions of primary health care nurses. **R. Pesq.: Cuid. Fundam. Online**, v. 13, p. 1186-1192, 2021. Available at https://seer.unirio.br/cuidadofundamental/article/view/9239/10172. Accessed on: 2 August 2024.

SOUZA, T. de C.; MONTEIRO, D. da R.; TREVISAN, B. F.; MALLMANN, F. H. Performance
nursing in the care of breast cancer patients: integrative review. **Research, Society and Development**, v. 9, n. 12, e14391210939, 2020. Available at: https://rsdjournal.org/index.php/rsd/article/view/10939/9758. Accessed on: 2 Aug. 2024.
STUMM, E. M. F.; LEITE, M. T.; MASCHIO, G. Experiences of a nursing team in caring for cancer patients. **Cogitare Enfermagem**, Curitiba, v.

13, n . 1 , p . 75-82, jan.-mar. 2018.Available at:
https://www.redalyc.org/pdf/4836/483648978010.pdf. Accessed on: 2 August 2024.

TEIXEIRA, M. de S.; GOLDMAN, R. E.; GONÇALVES, V. C. S.; GUTIÉRREZ, M. G.
R. de; FIGUEIREDO, E. N. de. The role of primary care nurses in breast cancer control. **Acta Paulista de Enfermagem**, São Paulo, v. 30, n. 1, p. 1-7, 2017.Available at:
https://www.scielo.br/j/ape/a/CPVVWkZg9Skpmcy6cczWFbv/?lang=pt&format=pdf. Accessed on: 2 August 2024.

URRÚTIA, G.; BONFILL, X. PRISMA statement: a proposal to improve the publication of systematic reviews and metaanalyses. **Med Clin (Barc)**, v.135, n.11, p.507-511, 2010.

VILLAR, R. R.; FERNÁNDEZ, S. P.; GAREA, C. C.; PILLADO, M. T. S.; BARREIRO,V. B.; MARTÍN, C. G. Quality of life and anxiety in women with breast cancer before and after treatment. **Latin American Journal of Nursing**, v. 25,art.e2958,2017.Availableat:
https://www.scielo.br/j/rlae/a/b4kQpywJX5jPstMFnGypfGN/?lang=pt&format=pdf.Accessed on: 30 July 2024.

WUNDER, A. P.; NORO, A.; REYES, V. B.; TIGRE, A.; CAVEDINI, T. V.; FILIPPON,D. C. C. Nursing consultation in the chemotherapy outpatient clinic: an experience report. **Semana de Enfermagem**, v. 28, p. 40, 2017.

ZINHANI, M. C. Prevention of cervical and breast cancer in a municipality in southern Brazil. **Arq. Catarin Meda**, v.47, n.2, p.23-34, 2018.

AUTHORS' BIOGRAPHIES

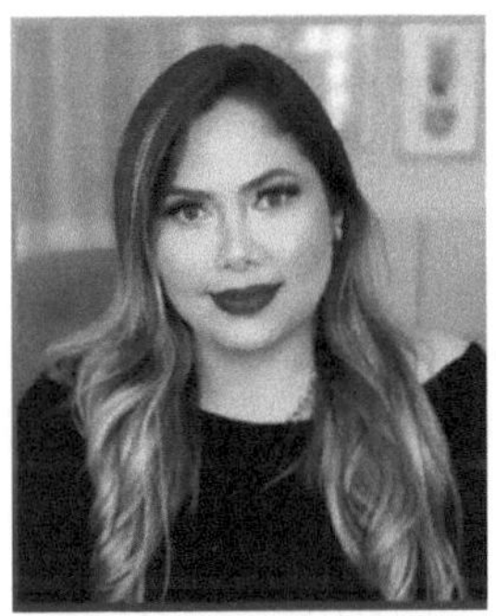

FABRIANE SOUSA ARAÚJO LIMA

Graduated in Nursing with a Bachelor's Degree from Santa Luzia College (FSL). Expertise in primary care and the hospital sector. Research in health.

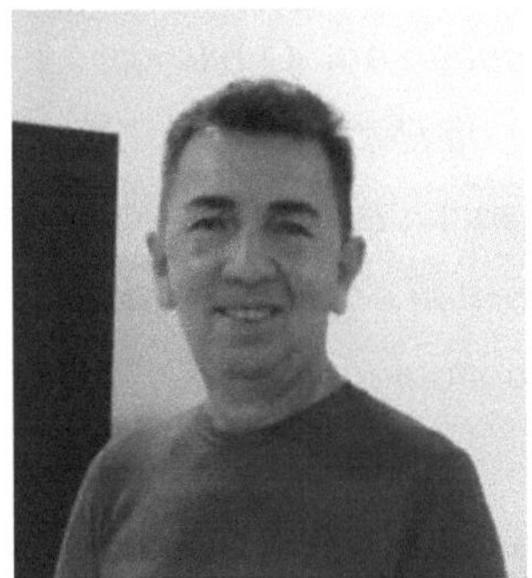

ANTONIO DA COSTA CARDOSO NETO

Post-Doctorate in Psychology from the University of Flores - Buenos Aires / Argentina (2023). PhD in Collective Health from the Federal University of Maranhão - UFMA (2021). PhD in Public Health Sciences from the University of Business and Social Sciences - UCES, Buenos Aires / Argentina (2018). Specialist in School Administration from the Cândido Mendes University, Rio de Janeiro (2010). Specialist in Elderly Health from Estácio de Sá University, Rio de Janeiro (2011). Graduated in Bachelor's Nursing from the Universidade CEUMA / MA (2008). Graduated in Pedagogy from the State University of Maranhão - UEMA (2001). He is the Coordinator of Postgraduate Research and Extension, Professor of Scientific Methodology and Member of the Structuring Teaching Centre of the Nursing course at Faculdade Santa Luzia -FSL (2017 - current), a teacher of Basic Education in the public education network of the Municipality of Santa Inês/Maranhão (1998 - current). He has been Coordinator of the Undergraduate Nursing Course since its creation (2012-2018), Academic Director (2018-2023), Institutional Prosecutor (PI) (2017-2023) and Institutional Researcher -CENSUP (2018) at Faculdade Santa Luzia - FSL. He was coordinator and teacher of technical courses at the Santa Luzia Technical School of Commerce - ETCSL / Maranhão (1996-2017). Assistant researcher at the Federal University of Maranhão - UFMA (2006-2008). Researcher and Principal Sponsor of the Project: Biopsychosocial Education and Quality of Life for the Elderly. Has experience in drawing up Pedagogical Projects for Undergraduate Courses and drawing up Institutional Development Plans (PDI) Contact: (098) 981090921. E-mail address:cardosoneto.acc@gmail.com; cardosonetofsl2018@outlook.com.br. ORCID: https://orcid.org/0000-0003-3771-2821

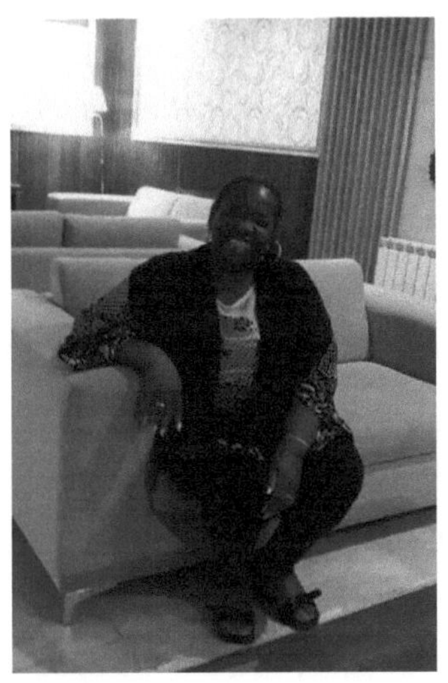

MARCIA SILVA DE OLIVEIRA

Post-Doctorate in Psychology - University of Flores (UFLO), Argentina. PhD in Public Health Sciences - Universidad de Ciencias Empresariales y Sociales (UCES), Argentina. Collaborating researcher at CITAB - Centre for Research and Agro-environmental and Biological Technologies at the University of Trás-os-Montes and Alto Douro/Portugal. Master in Health SciencesUniversity of Brasília (UnB). Postgraduate in Clinical Analyses (Cytopathology)São Judas Tadeu College/RJ. Postgraduate Degree in Pathology - Castelo Branco University/RJ. Postgraduate in University Teaching (Research Methodology and Pedagogical Research and Practice) - UniCEUB/DF. Graduated in Biological Sciences - Medical Modality (Biomedicine) from the State University of Rio de Janeiro (Anatomy). General/Pedagogical Coordinator of the Brasília Campus of Universidade Paulista (UNIP/Brasília). Lecturer in Pathology, Immunology, Didactics Applied to Nursing, Educational Practice in Health and Integrating Seminar on the Nursing course at Faculdade Santa Luzia (FSL)/Santa Inês/MA. Lecturer with experience in organising, participating in, coordinating, planning and monitoring health and education projects, both inside and outside pedagogical learning spaces. Good interpersonal relationships, responsibility and dedication to work activities. Biomedical Supervisor at Laboratório Médico Dr Maricondi Ltda (WAMA Diagnóstica), São Carlos/SP (Costa Verde Unit - Itaguaí/RJ). Lecturer in Safety, Environment and Health and Quality Management Systems at the Rio de Janeiro State Technical School Support Foundation (FAETEC/RJ).

Professor of Medicine, Dentistry, Nursing, Veterinary Medicine and Architecture and Urbanism at the Faculdades Integradas do Planalto Central (FACIPLAC/DF). Lecturer on undergraduate courses in Biomedicine, Physiotherapy, Psychology, Biological Sciences and Maths at Universidade Paulista (UNIP - Campus Brasília). Coordinator and lecturer on postgraduate and extension courses at the Evangelical Educational Institute of the Centre-West - UNIECO/DF. Lecturer in Hormonology on the Postgraduate course in Clinical, Toxicological and Bromatological Analyses at the Instituto Brasil Pesquisa e Extensão - IBEP. Full Researcher at the Centre for Health Promotion Studies and Inclusive Projects at the University of Brasilia - NESPROM/UnB.

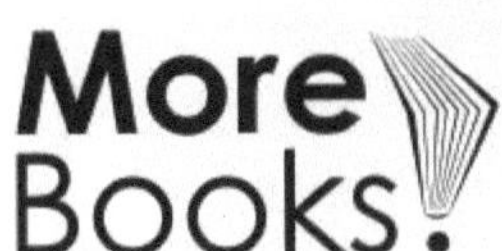

I want morebooks!

Buy your books fast and straightforward online - at one of world's fastest growing online book stores! Environmentally sound due to Print-on-Demand technologies.

Buy your books online at
www.morebooks.shop

Kaufen Sie Ihre Bücher schnell und unkompliziert online – auf einer der am schnellsten wachsenden Buchhandelsplattformen weltweit! Dank Print-On-Demand umwelt- und ressourcenschonend produziert.

Bücher schneller online kaufen
www.morebooks.shop

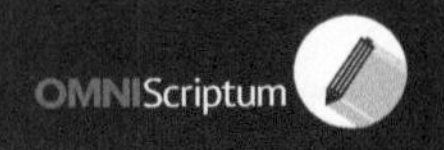

Printed by Books on Demand GmbH, Norderstedt / Germany